WordTOOLS For Self Esteem

Vol. 1

Harnessing the
Power of Words!

Carol L Rickard, LCSW

Well YOUniversity® Publications

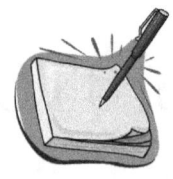

Sign up now!

To be sure to get our weekly motivational & inspirational quotes and stories!

ThePowerOfWordsEQuote.com

Copyright © 2017 Carol L. Rickard

All Licensing by Well YOUniversity, LLC

All rights reserved.

ISBN-13: 978-1-947745-06-3

WordTools for Self Esteem Vol. 1

Harnessing the Power of Words!

by Carol L Rickard, LCSW

© Copyright 2017 Well YOUniversity Publications

ISBN 13: 978-1-947745-06-3

All rights reserved.

No part of this book may be reproduced for resale, redistribution, or any other purposes (including but not limited to eBooks, pamphlets, articles, video or audiotapes, & handouts or slides for lectures or workshops).

Licenses to reproduce these materials for those and any other purposes must be obtained from the author and Well YOUniversity.

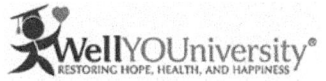

888 LIFE TOOLS (543-3866)

Carol@WellYOUniversity.com

Welcome!

My 1st WordTool came to me in 2006 when doing a group with my patients. How could I get them to w*elcome* change in their lives?

Creating **H**ealthy **A**nd **N**ew **G**rowth **E**xperiences!

From there it's been an onward journey! Most of them are inspired by persons or situations. All of them I use in my own life. My hope is to create Ah-Ah moments that can help change a life!

They are officially called "Artinyms", which is Sanskrit for "describe".

On the back of each wordtool is a question for you. Answering them will serve to strengthen and build your self-esteem from the inside out!

~To Living Well TODAY! ~

Carol

ACCEPT	1	FORGIVE	31
ACTION	3	GRATEFUL	33
ASK	5	IMPACT	35
AWARE	7	LIFE	37
BELIEFS	9	LOVE	39
BLAME	11	PAST	41
CHAOS	13	PEACE	43
COMMIT	15	PURPOSE	45
COURAGE	17	REFLECT	47
DISCIPLINE	19	SERVE	49
DOUBT	21	SHAME	51
DREAM	23	STIGMA	53
EMOTION	25	SURRENDER	55
EXCUSE	27	TOXIC	57
FEEL	29	URGES	59

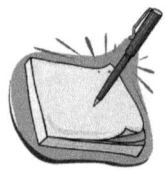

Sign up now!

To be sure to get our weekly motivational & inspirational quotes and stories!

ThePowerOfWordsEQuote.com

A

Conscious

Choice

Enabling

Powerful

Transformation

COPYRIGHT 2017 & Licensed by Well YOUniversity, LLC

What is something you struggle to *accept* that is holding you back from strengthening self esteem?

A

Critical

Task

Implemented

Only

Now!

COPYRIGHT 2017 & Licensed by Well YOUniversity, LLC

What *actions* are you taking to grow your self-esteem? What actions are hurting it?

Acquire

Self

Knowledge

COPYRIGHT 2017 & Licensed by Well YOUniversity, LLC

What is something you have been afraid to **ask**? Why? What's the impact on your self-esteem?

Actively

Work

At

Recognizing

Existence

COPYRIGHT 2017 & Licensed by Well YOUniversity, LLC

How would your life be different if you were more *aware* every day of what helps & hurts your self-esteem?

Binding

Energy

Linking

Intention

Everyday &

Finding

Success

COPYRIGHT 2017 & Licensed by Well YOUniversity, LLC

What negative *beliefs* are holding you back?
Where did they come from?

Become

Lost

Amongst

Many

Excuses!

COPYRIGHT 2017 & Licensed by Well YOUniversity, LLC

Who do you currently *blame* for the negative circumstances going on in your life?
How is this helping you?

Constantly

Having

Activity

Obstruct

Success!

COPYRIGHT 2017 & Licensed by Well YOUniversity, LLC

What would your self-esteem be if you were to get rid of some of the **chaos** in your life? What chaos do you need to get rid of?

Challenge

Ourselves

Make

Matters

Important

Today!

COPYRIGHT 2017 & Licensed by Well YOUniversity, LLC

What can you **commit** to that can help strengthen your self-esteem? Working on health? Relationships? Work?

Challenge

Ourselves

Under

Real

Adversity

Gaining

Empowerment

COPYRIGHT 2017 & Licensed by Well YOUniversity, LLC

When was the last time you called on *courage* to deal with a life situation? What was the outcome?

Deciding

I

Stay

Committed

In

Purpose

Letting

In

No

Excuse!

COPYRIGHT 2017 & Licensed by Well YOUniversity, LLC

Is there anything in your life you currently have ***discipline*** about? What do you think stops you from being more disciplined?

Dwell

On

Unfounded

Beliefs &

Thoughts!

COPYRIGHT 2017 & Licensed by Well YOUniversity, LLC

What are some of your **doubts** that could be holding you back? What would your life & self-esteem be like if they were not there?

Daringly

Recognize

Experiences

As

Mine!

COPYRIGHT 2017 & Licensed by Well YOUniversity, LLC

What are some of your *dreams*? Write them down here & visualize them happening every night before you fall asleep!

Energy

Matching

Our

Thoughts &

Influencing

Outcomes

Naturally

COPYRIGHT 2017 & Licensed by Well YOUniversity, LLC

How has *emotion* negatively impacted on your life? What emotions are the hardest for you to manage in a positive way?

Engage

Xternal

Circumstances

Undermining

Self

Empowerment

COPYRIGHT 2017 & Licensed by Well YOUniversity, LLC

Do you tend to be someone who uses **excuses?**
How do you think they have hurt or helped you?

Fully

Examine

Emotional

Lessons

COPYRIGHT 2017 & Licensed by Well YOUniversity, LLC

What are some of the ways you avoid having to *feel*? Do you eat? Use substances? Avoid? What have been the – consequences doing this?

Find

Ourselves

Releasing

Grievances

Including

Victim

Experiences

COPYRIGHT 2017 & Licensed by Well YOUniversity, LLC

What does this word mean to you? What do you need to **forgive** yourself for? How can your life be different if you 'release' what you're holding?

Giving

Respect

And

Thanks

Everyday

For

Unbelievable

Life!

COPYRIGHT 2017 & Licensed by Well YOUniversity, LLC

Make a list of all the things you are *grateful* for having in your life (minimum 30 things!) This includes little things too!

I

Make

Powerful

Adjustments

Concerning

Today!

COPYRIGHT 2017 & Licensed by Well YOUniversity, LLC

What are some behaviors having a negative effect on your self-esteem. What *impact* can you start to have & change this around?

Living

Intentionally &

Fully

Engaged

COPYRIGHT 2017 & Licensed by Well YOUniversity, LLC

What are some of the ways in which you are present in *life*? In other words, living intentionally & fully engaged!

Letting

Our

Vulnerabilities

Exist

COPYRIGHT 2017 & Licensed by Well YOUniversity, LLC

Who do you let yourself *feel* love for and why?
In other words, let your vulnerabilities show!

Powerful

Alignment

Sabotaging

Today

COPYRIGHT 2017 & Licensed by Well YOUniversity, LLC

What are some things from the **past** you need to let go of in order to strengthen your self-esteem?

Purposeful

Emotion

Allowing

Calm

Existence

COPYRIGHT 2017 & Licensed by Well YOUniversity, LLC

What are healthy ways you can create some *peace* in your life today?

Powerful

Underlying

Reason

Push

Ourselves

Stretch

Everyday

COPYRIGHT 2017 & Licensed by Well YOUniversity, LLC

What gives you **purpose**? If you're not sure, what are some things that are important to you? Can you use these for purpose?

Re-examine

Experiences

For

Lessons

Enabling

Correction

Today

COPYRIGHT 2017 & Licensed by Well YOUniversity, LLC

If you were to *reflect* on some times in your life where things either went well or didn't go so well, what are you able to learn from them?

See

Everyone

Receives

Valued

Existence

COPYRIGHT 2017 & Licensed by Well YOUniversity, LLC

What are some of the ways you *serve* others? In other words, how do you show people around you that you value their presence in your life?

Strongly

Held

Assumption

Minimizing

Existence

COPYRIGHT 2017 & Licensed by Well YOUniversity, LLC

Do you struggle with *shame?* If so, how do you think it impacts your self-esteem?

Strong

Thoughts

Influencing

Greatly

My

Acceptance

COPYRIGHT 2017 & Licensed by Well YOUniversity, LLC

Has *stigma* ever stopped you from asking for help or letting people know things about you? How do you think this has impacted your self-esteem?

Start

Unconditionally

Releasing &

Relinquishing

Expectations

N*ow*

Delivering

Empowerment &

Relief

COPYRIGHT 2017 & Licensed by Well YOUniversity, LLC

What are some areas in your life that are holding you hostage? How does this effect your self-esteem? What stops you from **surrendering**?

Take

Our

Xistence

Instead

Contributing

COPYRIGHT 2017 & Licensed by Well YOUniversity, LLC

How have *toxic* people impacted your self-esteem? Who or what toxic situations do you need to remove from your life?

Unstoppable

Responses

Greatly

Endangering

Self

COPYRIGHT 2017 & Licensed by Well YOUniversity, LLC

What are some of the negative behaviors that show up as *urges* in your life? How do they impact your self-esteem? What can life be like without them?

About the Author

Carol L Rickard, LCSW, TTS, of Hopewell, NJ is founder & CEO of WellYOUniversity, LLC, a global health education company dedicated *to empowering individuals with the tools and supports to achieve lifelong wellness & recovery.*

Also known as **America's Wellness Ambassador**, Carol is a dynamic & engaging speaker who brings to life practical / useful solutions. She is a weekly contributor for Esperanza Magazine; written 13 books on stress and wellness, had a guest appearance on Dr. Oz last year

She is also the creator & host of a 30-minute wellness show on Princeton TV - **The WELL YOU Show** which current episodes are aired on Mondays at 6:00pm EST & Sundays at 8:30am EST and can be watched at PrincetonTV.org.

All episodes available at: **www.TheWELLYOUShow.com**

Get more of Carol at:

Twitter: **@wellYOUlife**

"Like us" @ www.FaceBook.com/WellYOUniversity

Have Carol Speak at Your Next Event!

Get more information about how you can have Carol speak at your organization, event, or conference.

Go to: www.CarolLRickard.com

Or call: 888 Life Tools (543-3866)

Carol's Other Books

Getting Your Mind to Mind You
ANGER – A Simple & Practical Approach
Help – How to Help Those Who DON'T Want it
Selfness – Simple Self-Care Secrets
Stress Eating – How to STOP Using Food to Cope
Stretched Not Broken – Caregiver's Stress
The Caregiver's Toolbox
Transforming Illness to Wellness
Putting Your Weight Loss on Auto
The Benefits of Smoking
Moving Beyond Depression
LifeTools – How to Manage Life
Creating Compliance
Relapse Prevention

Please visit us at:

www.WellYOUniversity.com

Sign up for weekly motivational e-quote!

Check out our upcoming FREE webinars!

Learn more about our training programs.

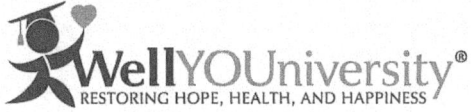

Email us your success story at:

Success@WellYOUniversity.com

We'd like to ask for your feedback

Please check out the next page
if this book has been HELPFUL for you!

We'd love to hear from you!

Feedback Card

Please take a moment & provide us some feedback about the book you just read & how you feel *it benefited YOU!*

Tear along here

_____

_____

_____

_____

Name: _____

Best Phone #: _____

Can we use your comments in our publicity materials?

Yes / No

If OK with you, what's the best time to call you:_____

Thank You!

Scan or take a picture & email:
Carol@WellYOUniversity.com

Snail mail: Carol Rickard
5 Zion Rd., Hopewell, NJ 08535

www.ingramcontent.com/pod-product-compliance
Lightning Source LLC
LaVergne TN
LVHW051209080426
835512LV00019B/3177